The Caregiver's Companion

Name of Caregiver

Name of Loved One(s)

Year

Goal for this Year

Published by The Chronic Creator Co. © 2024 Rachel C. Hill
Printed October 2024

No part of this book may be reproduced or transmitted in any form or by any means, electronic or mechanical, including photocopying and recording, or by any information storage or retrieval system, except as may be expressly permitted in writing by the publisher, Rachel Hill.

ISBN: 979-8-9913871-4-9

A Note from The Chronic Creator

Your role as a caregiver is incredibly important, and it often goes unnoticed. I want you to know that your efforts make a profound difference in the lives of those you care for.

Caring for someone has moments that can be both rewarding and challenging. It requires immense patience, compassion, and strength—qualities that you embody every day. Please remember that it's okay to take a step back and acknowledge your own feelings. Caring for others is a beautiful gift, but it can also be overwhelming at times. Don't hesitate to reach out to your support network when you need it.

Take time for yourself, even if it's just a few quiet moments with a book or a walk outside. Self-care isn't selfish; it's essential for your well-being. You can't pour from an empty cup, and your health—both physical and emotional—matters deeply.

Every act of kindness you show, no matter how small, creates a ripple effect of positivity. You are not just providing care; you are offering love, comfort, and dignity to those who need it most. Remember that your hard work does not go unnoticed, and the impact you have is far-reaching.

Stay strong and take pride in the incredible work you do. You are making a difference every day, and that is something to celebrate.

With gratitude and encouragement,
The Chronic Creator

@thechroniccreatorco   thechroniccreatorco@gmail.com   thechroniccreatorco.etsy.com

Basic Information

Personal Information

Name		DOB	
Phone		Gender	
Address			
Email		Blood Type	
Main Illness(es)			
Allergies			

Emergency Contact Information

Name		Relationship	
Phone		Alt. Phone	
Email			
Additional Notes			

Secondary Emergency Contact Information

Name		Relationship	
Phone		Alt. Phone	
Email			
Additional Notes			

Medical History

Date	Diagnosis, Surgery, Hospitalization, Etc.	Notes

Health Insurance Information

Provider			
Policy #		Group #	
Claims Address		Insurance Phone #	
Additional Notes			

Medications

Medication or Supplement	Dosage	Reason for Taking	Notes

Mood Tracker

	Jan	Feb	Mar	April	May	June	July	Aug	Sept	Oct	Nov	Dec
1												
2												
3												
4												
5												
6												
7												
8												
9												
10												
11												
12												
13												
14												
15												
16												
17												
18												
19												
20												
21												
22												
23												
24												
25												
26												
27												
28												
29												
30												
31												

Key

☐
☐
☐
☐
☐
☐

You'll never know how much your caring matters.

Note to Self

Write an encouraging letter or note to yourself for the hard days.

_____
_____
_____
_____
_____
_____
_____
_____
_____
_____
_____
_____
_____
_____
_____
_____

Lab Results

Date	Labs Run	Results

Medical Contacts

Specialty:			
Doctor's Name		Office Name	
Email		Phone	
Address			
Additional Notes			

Specialty:			
Doctor's Name		Office Name	
Email		Phone	
Address			
Additional Notes			

Specialty:			
Doctor's Name		Office Name	
Email		Phone	
Address			
Additional Notes			

Medical Contacts

Specialty:			
Doctor's Name		Office Name	
Email		Phone	
Address			
Additional Notes			

Specialty:			
Doctor's Name		Office Name	
Email		Phone	
Address			
Additional Notes			

Specialty:			
Doctor's Name		Office Name	
Email		Phone	
Address			
Additional Notes			

Medical Contacts

Specialty:			
Doctor's Name		Office Name	
Email		Phone	
Address			
Additional Notes			

Specialty:			
Doctor's Name		Office Name	
Email		Phone	
Address			
Additional Notes			

Specialty:			
Doctor's Name		Office Name	
Email		Phone	
Address			
Additional Notes			

Medical Contacts

Specialty:			
Doctor's Name		Office Name	
Email		Phone	
Address			
Additional Notes			

Specialty:			
Doctor's Name		Office Name	
Email		Phone	
Address			
Additional Notes			

Specialty:			
Doctor's Name		Office Name	
Email		Phone	
Address			
Additional Notes			

Legal and Financial Contacts

Specialty:			
Name		Office/Firm Name	
Email		Phone	
Address			
Additional Notes			

Specialty:			
Name		Office/Firm Name	
Email		Phone	
Address			
Additional Notes			

Specialty:			
Name		Office/Firm Name	
Email		Phone	
Address			
Additional Notes			

Appointment Logs

Doctor Seen		**Date & Time**	
Reason for Visit		**Next Appt.**	
Questions or Concerns			
Doctor's Notes			
Key Takeaways			

Doctor Seen		**Date & Time**	
Reason for Visit		**Next Appt.**	
Questions or Concerns			
Doctor's Notes			
Key Takeaways			

Appointment Logs

Doctor Seen		**Date & Time**	
Reason for Visit		**Next Appt.**	
Questions or Concerns			
Doctor's Notes			
Key Takeaways			

Doctor Seen		**Date & Time**	
Reason for Visit		**Next Appt.**	
Questions or Concerns			
Doctor's Notes			
Key Takeaways			

Appointment Logs

Doctor Seen		**Date & Time**	
Reason for Visit		**Next Appt.**	
Questions or Concerns			
Doctor's Notes			
Key Takeaways			

Doctor Seen		**Date & Time**	
Reason for Visit		**Next Appt.**	
Questions or Concerns			
Doctor's Notes			
Key Takeaways			

Appointment Logs

Doctor Seen		Date & Time	
Reason for Visit		Next Appt.	
Questions or Concerns			
Doctor's Notes			
Key Takeaways			

Doctor Seen		Date & Time	
Reason for Visit		Next Appt.	
Questions or Concerns			
Doctor's Notes			
Key Takeaways			

Appointment Logs

Doctor Seen		Date & Time	
Reason for Visit		Next Appt.	
Questions or Concerns			
Doctor's Notes			
Key Takeaways			

Doctor Seen		Date & Time	
Reason for Visit		Next Appt.	
Questions or Concerns			
Doctor's Notes			
Key Takeaways			

Important Upcoming Dates

Date	Important Event	Notes

Important Upcoming Dates

Date	Important Event	Notes

Treatments Tried

Date	Treatment	Results	Notes

Next Steps

Treatment to Try	Intended Results	Notes

Food Sensitivity Tracker

Use this page to keep track of foods that are safe and enjoyable for your loved one(s) to eat and which foods to avoid based on symptoms, allergies, or tastes.

Safe Foods	Okay in Moderation	Foods to Avoid

Vaccinations and Shots

Date	Vaccination or Shot	Notes

Medical Expenses Tracker

Date	Description	Total Billed	Covered by Insurance	Balance Due	Paid?
		Total			

Yearly Medical Overview

January	February	March

April	May	June

July	August	September

October	November	December

Top 5 Goals for the Year

Notes

Notes

Notes

Notes

Notes

January

YEAR: _____

SUNDAY	MONDAY	TUESDAY	WEDNESDAY	THURSDAY	FRIDAY	SATURDAY

Habit Tracker

Month		Year	

HABIT	1	2	3	4	5	6	7	8	9	10	11	12	13	14	15	16	17	18	19	20	21	22	23	24	25	26	27	28	29	30	31

Symptom Tracker

SYMPTOM	1	2	3	4	5	6	7	8	9	10	11	12	13	14	15	16	17	18	19	20	21	22	23	24	25	26	27	28	29	30	31

WEEKLY
planner

WEEK OF _____

MONDAY

TUESDAY

WEDNESDAY

THURSDAY

FRIDAY

SATURDAY

SUNDAY

Notes

PRIORITIES

WEEKLY
planner WEEK OF _____

MONDAY

TUESDAY

WEDNESDAY

THURSDAY

FRIDAY

SATURDAY

SUNDAY

Notes

PRIORITIES

WEEKLY
planner

WEEK OF _____

Notes

PRIORITIES

- MONDAY
- TUESDAY
- WEDNESDAY
- THURSDAY
- FRIDAY
- SATURDAY
- SUNDAY

WEEKLY
planner

WEEK OF _____

MONDAY

TUESDAY

WEDNESDAY

THURSDAY

FRIDAY

SATURDAY

SUNDAY

Notes

PRIORITIES

WEEKLY
planner

WEEK OF _____

MONDAY

TUESDAY

WEDNESDAY

THURSDAY

FRIDAY

SATURDAY

SUNDAY

Notes

PRIORITIES

MONTH:

REVIEW

ILLNESS MANAGEMENT ★ ★ ★ ★ ★   MOOD ★ ★ ★ ★ ★

HIGHLIGHTS OF THE MONTH

THINGS I LEARNED

THINGS I'M GRATEFUL FOR

WAYS TO IMPROVE NEXT MONTH

February

YEAR: _____

SUNDAY	MONDAY	TUESDAY	WEDNESDAY	THURSDAY	FRIDAY	SATURDAY

Habit Tracker

| Month | | Year | |

HABIT	1	2	3	4	5	6	7	8	9	10	11	12	13	14	15	16	17	18	19	20	21	22	23	24	25	26	27	28	29	30	31

Symptom Tracker

SYMPTOM	1	2	3	4	5	6	7	8	9	10	11	12	13	14	15	16	17	18	19	20	21	22	23	24	25	26	27	28	29	30	31

WEEKLY
planner

WEEK OF _____

MONDAY

TUESDAY

WEDNESDAY

THURSDAY

FRIDAY

SATURDAY

SUNDAY

Notes

PRIORITIES

○ _____
○ _____
○ _____
○ _____
○ _____
○ _____
○ _____
○ _____

WEEKLY
planner

WEEK OF _____

Notes

_____
_____
_____
_____
_____
_____
_____
_____
_____
_____
_____
_____
_____
_____
_____

MONDAY

TUESDAY

WEDNESDAY

THURSDAY

FRIDAY

SATURDAY

SUNDAY

PRIORITIES

○ _____
○ _____
○ _____
○ _____
○ _____
○ _____
○ _____
○ _____

WEEKLY
planner

WEEK OF _____

MONDAY

TUESDAY

WEDNESDAY

THURSDAY

FRIDAY

SATURDAY

SUNDAY

Notes

PRIORITIES

WEEKLY
planner

WEEK OF _____

MONDAY

TUESDAY

WEDNESDAY

THURSDAY

FRIDAY

SATURDAY

SUNDAY

Notes

_____
_____
_____
_____
_____
_____
_____
_____
_____
_____
_____
_____
_____
_____

PRIORITIES

○ _____
○ _____
○ _____
○ _____
○ _____
○ _____
○ _____
○ _____

WEEKLY *planner*

WEEK OF _____

MONDAY

TUESDAY

WEDNESDAY

THURSDAY

FRIDAY

SATURDAY

SUNDAY

Notes

PRIORITIES

MONTH:

REVIEW

ILLNESS MANAGEMENT ★★★★★   MOOD ★★★★★

HIGHLIGHTS OF THE MONTH

THINGS I LEARNED

THINGS I'M GRATEFUL FOR

WAYS TO IMPROVE NEXT MONTH

March

YEAR: _____

SUNDAY	MONDAY	TUESDAY	WEDNESDAY	THURSDAY	FRIDAY	SATURDAY

Habit Tracker

Month		Year	

HABIT	1	2	3	4	5	6	7	8	9	10	11	12	13	14	15	16	17	18	19	20	21	22	23	24	25	26	27	28	29	30	31

Symptom Tracker

SYMPTOM	1	2	3	4	5	6	7	8	9	10	11	12	13	14	15	16	17	18	19	20	21	22	23	24	25	26	27	28	29	30	31

WEEKLY
planner

WEEK OF _____

MONDAY	
TUESDAY	
WEDNESDAY	
THURSDAY	
FRIDAY	
SATURDAY	
SUNDAY	

Notes

PRIORITIES

- ○
- ○
- ○
- ○
- ○
- ○
- ○
- ○

WEEKLY *planner*

WEEK OF _____

MONDAY	
TUESDAY	
WEDNESDAY	
THURSDAY	
FRIDAY	
SATURDAY	
SUNDAY	

Notes

_____
_____
_____
_____
_____
_____
_____
_____
_____
_____
_____
_____
_____
_____
_____

PRIORITIES

○ _____
○ _____
○ _____
○ _____
○ _____
○ _____
○ _____
○ _____

WEEKLY
planner

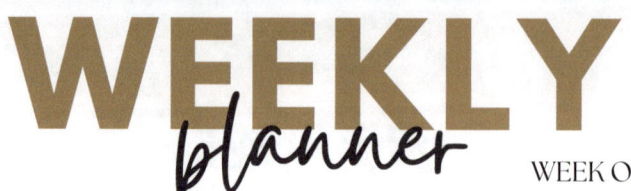

WEEK OF _____

MONDAY

TUESDAY

WEDNESDAY

THURSDAY

FRIDAY

SATURDAY

SUNDAY

Notes

_____
_____
_____
_____
_____
_____
_____
_____
_____
_____
_____
_____
_____
_____
_____
_____

PRIORITIES

○ _____
○ _____
○ _____
○ _____
○ _____
○ _____
○ _____
○ _____

WEEKLY
planner WEEK OF _____

MONDAY

TUESDAY

WEDNESDAY

THURSDAY

FRIDAY

SATURDAY

SUNDAY

Notes

PRIORITIES

WEEKLY
planner

WEEK OF _____

MONDAY

TUESDAY

WEDNESDAY

THURSDAY

FRIDAY

SATURDAY

SUNDAY

Notes

_____
_____
_____
_____
_____
_____
_____
_____
_____
_____
_____
_____
_____
_____

PRIORITIES

○ _____
○ _____
○ _____
○ _____
○ _____
○ _____
○ _____
○ _____

MONTH: REVIEW

ILLNESS MANAGEMENT ★ ★ ★ ★ ★   MOOD ★ ★ ★ ★ ★

HIGHLIGHTS OF THE MONTH

THINGS I LEARNED

THINGS I'M GRATEFUL FOR

WAYS TO IMPROVE NEXT MONTH

April

YEAR: _____

SUNDAY	MONDAY	TUESDAY	WEDNESDAY	THURSDAY	FRIDAY	SATURDAY

Habit Tracker

Month		Year	

HABIT	1	2	3	4	5	6	7	8	9	10	11	12	13	14	15	16	17	18	19	20	21	22	23	24	25	26	27	28	29	30	31

Symptom Tracker

SYMPTOM	1	2	3	4	5	6	7	8	9	10	11	12	13	14	15	16	17	18	19	20	21	22	23	24	25	26	27	28	29	30	31

WEEKLY
planner

WEEK OF _____

MONDAY

TUESDAY

WEDNESDAY

THURSDAY

FRIDAY

SATURDAY

SUNDAY

Notes
_____
_____
_____
_____
_____
_____
_____
_____
_____
_____
_____
_____
_____
_____
_____
_____
_____
_____

PRIORITIES
○ _____
○ _____
○ _____
○ _____
○ _____
○ _____
○ _____
○ _____

WEEKLY
planner

WEEK OF _____

- MONDAY
- TUESDAY
- WEDNESDAY
- THURSDAY
- FRIDAY
- SATURDAY
- SUNDAY

Notes

PRIORITIES

WEEKLY
planner

WEEK OF _____

Notes

MONDAY

TUESDAY

WEDNESDAY

THURSDAY

FRIDAY

SATURDAY

SUNDAY

PRIORITIES
- ○
- ○
- ○
- ○
- ○
- ○
- ○
- ○

WEEKLY
planner

WEEK OF _____

MONDAY

TUESDAY

WEDNESDAY

THURSDAY

FRIDAY

SATURDAY

SUNDAY

Notes

PRIORITIES

○ _____
○ _____
○ _____
○ _____
○ _____
○ _____
○ _____
○ _____

WEEKLY
planner

WEEK OF _____

MONDAY	
TUESDAY	
WEDNESDAY	
THURSDAY	
FRIDAY	
SATURDAY	
SUNDAY	

Notes

_____
_____
_____
_____
_____
_____
_____
_____
_____
_____
_____
_____
_____
_____
_____
_____
_____

PRIORITIES

○ _____
○ _____
○ _____
○ _____
○ _____
○ _____
○ _____
○ _____

MONTH: REVIEW

ILLNESS MANAGEMENT ★ ★ ★ ★ ★   **MOOD** ★ ★ ★ ★ ★

HIGHLIGHTS OF THE MONTH

THINGS I LEARNED

THINGS I'M GRATEFUL FOR

WAYS TO IMPROVE NEXT MONTH

May

YEAR: _____

SUNDAY	MONDAY	TUESDAY	WEDNESDAY	THURSDAY	FRIDAY	SATURDAY

Habit Tracker

| Month | | Year | |

HABIT	1	2	3	4	5	6	7	8	9	10	11	12	13	14	15	16	17	18	19	20	21	22	23	24	25	26	27	28	29	30	31

Symptom Tracker

SYMPTOM	1	2	3	4	5	6	7	8	9	10	11	12	13	14	15	16	17	18	19	20	21	22	23	24	25	26	27	28	29	30	31

WEEKLY *planner*

WEEK OF _____

MONDAY

TUESDAY

WEDNESDAY

THURSDAY

FRIDAY

SATURDAY

SUNDAY

Notes

_____
_____
_____
_____
_____
_____
_____
_____
_____
_____
_____
_____
_____
_____
_____

PRIORITIES

○ _____
○ _____
○ _____
○ _____
○ _____
○ _____
○ _____
○ _____

WEEKLY *planner*

WEEK OF _____

MONDAY

TUESDAY

WEDNESDAY

THURSDAY

FRIDAY

SATURDAY

SUNDAY

Notes

PRIORITIES

- ○
- ○
- ○
- ○
- ○
- ○
- ○
- ○
- ○

WEEKLY
planner

WEEK OF _____

MONDAY

TUESDAY

WEDNESDAY

THURSDAY

FRIDAY

SATURDAY

SUNDAY

Notes

_____
_____
_____
_____
_____
_____
_____
_____
_____
_____
_____
_____
_____
_____
_____
_____

PRIORITIES

○ _____
○ _____
○ _____
○ _____
○ _____
○ _____
○ _____
○ _____

WEEKLY
planner WEEK OF _____

MONDAY

TUESDAY

WEDNESDAY

THURSDAY

FRIDAY

SATURDAY

SUNDAY

Notes

PRIORITIES
- _____
- _____
- _____
- _____
- _____
- _____
- _____
- _____

WEEKLY
planner

WEEK OF _____

MONDAY

TUESDAY

WEDNESDAY

THURSDAY

FRIDAY

SATURDAY

SUNDAY

Notes

PRIORITIES

MONTH:

REVIEW

ILLNESS MANAGEMENT ★ ★ ★ ★ ★   MOOD ★ ★ ★ ★ ★

HIGHLIGHTS OF THE MONTH

THINGS I LEARNED

THINGS I'M GRATEFUL FOR

WAYS TO IMPROVE NEXT MONTH

June

YEAR: _____

SUNDAY	MONDAY	TUESDAY	WEDNESDAY	THURSDAY	FRIDAY	SATURDAY

Habit Tracker

| Month | | Year | |

HABIT	1	2	3	4	5	6	7	8	9	10	11	12	13	14	15	16	17	18	19	20	21	22	23	24	25	26	27	28	29	30	31

Symptom Tracker

SYMPTOM	1	2	3	4	5	6	7	8	9	10	11	12	13	14	15	16	17	18	19	20	21	22	23	24	25	26	27	28	29	30	31

WEEKLY
planner

WEEK OF _____

MONDAY

TUESDAY

WEDNESDAY

THURSDAY

FRIDAY

SATURDAY

SUNDAY

Notes

PRIORITIES

WEEKLY
planner

WEEK OF _____

MONDAY

TUESDAY

WEDNESDAY

THURSDAY

FRIDAY

SATURDAY

SUNDAY

Notes

PRIORITIES
- ○ _____
- ○ _____
- ○ _____
- ○ _____
- ○ _____
- ○ _____
- ○ _____
- ○ _____

WEEKLY
planner

WEEK OF _____

MONDAY

TUESDAY

WEDNESDAY

THURSDAY

FRIDAY

SATURDAY

SUNDAY

Notes

PRIORITIES

- ○
- ○
- ○
- ○
- ○
- ○
- ○
- ○

WEEKLY
planner

WEEK OF _____

MONDAY

TUESDAY

WEDNESDAY

THURSDAY

FRIDAY

SATURDAY

SUNDAY

Notes

PRIORITIES

WEEKLY
planner

WEEK OF _____

MONDAY

TUESDAY

WEDNESDAY

THURSDAY

FRIDAY

SATURDAY

SUNDAY

Notes

PRIORITIES

MONTH:

REVIEW

ILLNESS MANAGEMENT ★ ★ ★ ★ ★   MOOD ★ ★ ★ ★ ★

HIGHLIGHTS OF THE MONTH

THINGS I LEARNED

THINGS I'M GRATEFUL FOR

WAYS TO IMPROVE NEXT MONTH

July

YEAR: _____

SUNDAY	MONDAY	TUESDAY	WEDNESDAY	THURSDAY	FRIDAY	SATURDAY

Habit Tracker

| Month | | Year | |

HABIT	1	2	3	4	5	6	7	8	9	10	11	12	13	14	15	16	17	18	19	20	21	22	23	24	25	26	27	28	29	30	31

Symptom Tracker

SYMPTOM	1	2	3	4	5	6	7	8	9	10	11	12	13	14	15	16	17	18	19	20	21	22	23	24	25	26	27	28	29	30	31

WEEKLY
planner

WEEK OF _____

MONDAY

TUESDAY

WEDNESDAY

THURSDAY

FRIDAY

SATURDAY

SUNDAY

Notes

_____
_____
_____
_____
_____
_____
_____
_____
_____
_____
_____
_____
_____
_____
_____
_____
_____
_____

PRIORITIES

○ _____
○ _____
○ _____
○ _____
○ _____
○ _____
○ _____
○ _____
○ _____

WEEKLY
planner

WEEK OF _____

MONDAY

TUESDAY

WEDNESDAY

THURSDAY

FRIDAY

SATURDAY

SUNDAY

Notes

_____
_____
_____
_____
_____
_____
_____
_____
_____
_____
_____
_____
_____
_____
_____

PRIORITIES

○ _____
○ _____
○ _____
○ _____
○ _____
○ _____
○ _____
○ _____

WEEKLY
planner

WEEK OF _____

MONDAY

TUESDAY

WEDNESDAY

THURSDAY

FRIDAY

SATURDAY

SUNDAY

Notes

PRIORITIES

WEEKLY
planner

WEEK OF _____

MONDAY	
TUESDAY	
WEDNESDAY	
THURSDAY	
FRIDAY	
SATURDAY	
SUNDAY	

Notes

_____
_____
_____
_____
_____
_____
_____
_____
_____
_____
_____
_____
_____
_____
_____
_____
_____

PRIORITIES

○ _____
○ _____
○ _____
○ _____
○ _____
○ _____
○ _____
○ _____
○ _____

WEEKLY
planner

WEEK OF _____

MONDAY	
TUESDAY	
WEDNESDAY	
THURSDAY	
FRIDAY	
SATURDAY	
SUNDAY	

Notes
_____
_____
_____
_____
_____
_____
_____
_____
_____
_____
_____
_____
_____
_____

PRIORITIES
☐ _____
☐ _____
☐ _____
☐ _____
☐ _____
☐ _____
☐ _____
☐ _____
☐ _____

MONTH:

REVIEW

ILLNESS MANAGEMENT ★ ★ ★ ★ ★   MOOD ★ ★ ★ ★ ★

HIGHLIGHTS OF THE MONTH

THINGS I LEARNED

THINGS I'M GRATEFUL FOR

WAYS TO IMPROVE NEXT MONTH

August

YEAR:_____

SUNDAY	MONDAY	TUESDAY	WEDNESDAY	THURSDAY	FRIDAY	SATURDAY

Habit Tracker

Month		Year	

HABIT	1	2	3	4	5	6	7	8	9	10	11	12	13	14	15	16	17	18	19	20	21	22	23	24	25	26	27	28	29	30	31

Symptom Tracker

SYMPTOM	1	2	3	4	5	6	7	8	9	10	11	12	13	14	15	16	17	18	19	20	21	22	23	24	25	26	27	28	29	30	31

WEEKLY
planner

WEEK OF _____

MONDAY

TUESDAY

WEDNESDAY

THURSDAY

FRIDAY

SATURDAY

SUNDAY

Notes

PRIORITIES

WEEKLY
planner

WEEK OF _____

MONDAY

TUESDAY

WEDNESDAY

THURSDAY

FRIDAY

SATURDAY

SUNDAY

Notes

PRIORITIES

- ○ _____
- ○ _____
- ○ _____
- ○ _____
- ○ _____
- ○ _____
- ○ _____
- ○ _____

WEEKLY
planner

WEEK OF _____

MONDAY

TUESDAY

WEDNESDAY

THURSDAY

FRIDAY

SATURDAY

SUNDAY

Notes

_____
_____
_____
_____
_____
_____
_____
_____
_____
_____
_____
_____
_____
_____
_____

PRIORITIES

- ○ _____
- ○ _____
- ○ _____
- ○ _____
- ○ _____
- ○ _____
- ○ _____
- ○ _____

WEEKLY
planner

WEEK OF _____

MONDAY

TUESDAY

WEDNESDAY

THURSDAY

FRIDAY

SATURDAY

SUNDAY

Notes

PRIORITIES

WEEKLY
planner

WEEK OF _____

MONDAY

TUESDAY

WEDNESDAY

THURSDAY

FRIDAY

SATURDAY

SUNDAY

Notes

_____
_____
_____
_____
_____
_____
_____
_____
_____
_____
_____
_____
_____
_____
_____
_____

PRIORITIES

○ _____
○ _____
○ _____
○ _____
○ _____
○ _____
○ _____
○ _____

MONTH:

REVIEW

ILLNESS MANAGEMENT ★ ★ ★ ★ ★   MOOD ★ ★ ★ ★ ★

HIGHLIGHTS OF THE MONTH

THINGS I LEARNED

THINGS I'M GRATEFUL FOR

WAYS TO IMPROVE NEXT MONTH

September

YEAR:

SUNDAY	MONDAY	TUESDAY	WEDNESDAY	THURSDAY	FRIDAY	SATURDAY

Habit Tracker

| Month | | Year | |

HABIT	1	2	3	4	5	6	7	8	9	10	11	12	13	14	15	16	17	18	19	20	21	22	23	24	25	26	27	28	29	30	31

Symptom Tracker

SYMPTOM	1	2	3	4	5	6	7	8	9	10	11	12	13	14	15	16	17	18	19	20	21	22	23	24	25	26	27	28	29	30	31

WEEKLY
planner

WEEK OF _____

MONDAY

TUESDAY

WEDNESDAY

THURSDAY

FRIDAY

SATURDAY

SUNDAY

Notes

_____
_____
_____
_____
_____
_____
_____
_____
_____
_____
_____
_____
_____
_____
_____
_____
_____

PRIORITIES

○ _____
○ _____
○ _____
○ _____
○ _____
○ _____
○ _____
○ _____
○ _____

WEEKLY
planner WEEK OF _____

Notes

MONDAY

TUESDAY

WEDNESDAY

THURSDAY

FRIDAY

SATURDAY

SUNDAY

PRIORITIES

WEEKLY
planner

WEEK OF _____

MONDAY

TUESDAY

WEDNESDAY

THURSDAY

FRIDAY

SATURDAY

SUNDAY

Notes

_____
_____
_____
_____
_____
_____
_____
_____
_____
_____
_____
_____
_____
_____

PRIORITIES

○ _____
○ _____
○ _____
○ _____
○ _____
○ _____
○ _____
○ _____

WEEKLY
planner

WEEK OF _____

MONDAY	
TUESDAY	
WEDNESDAY	
THURSDAY	
FRIDAY	
SATURDAY	
SUNDAY	

Notes

PRIORITIES

WEEKLY
planner

WEEK OF _____

MONDAY

TUESDAY

WEDNESDAY

THURSDAY

FRIDAY

SATURDAY

SUNDAY

Notes

_____
_____
_____
_____
_____
_____
_____
_____
_____
_____
_____
_____
_____
_____
_____

PRIORITIES

○ _____
○ _____
○ _____
○ _____
○ _____
○ _____
○ _____
○ _____
○ _____

MONTH: REVIEW

ILLNESS MANAGEMENT ★ ★ ★ ★ ★   MOOD ★ ★ ★ ★ ★

HIGHLIGHTS OF THE MONTH

THINGS I LEARNED

THINGS I'M GRATEFUL FOR

WAYS TO IMPROVE NEXT MONTH

October

YEAR:

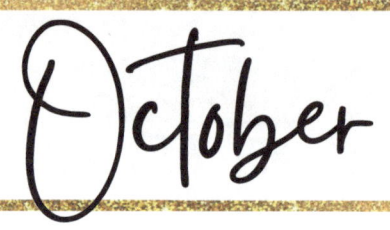

SUNDAY	MONDAY	TUESDAY	WEDNESDAY	THURSDAY	FRIDAY	SATURDAY

Habit Tracker

Month		Year	

HABIT	1	2	3	4	5	6	7	8	9	10	11	12	13	14	15	16	17	18	19	20	21	22	23	24	25	26	27	28	29	30	31

Symptom Tracker

SYMPTOM	1	2	3	4	5	6	7	8	9	10	11	12	13	14	15	16	17	18	19	20	21	22	23	24	25	26	27	28	29	30	31

WEEKLY
planner

WEEK OF _____

MONDAY

TUESDAY

WEDNESDAY

THURSDAY

FRIDAY

SATURDAY

SUNDAY

Notes

_____
_____
_____
_____
_____
_____
_____
_____
_____
_____
_____
_____
_____
_____

PRIORITIES

○ _____
○ _____
○ _____
○ _____
○ _____
○ _____
○ _____
○ _____

WEEKLY
planner WEEK OF _____

MONDAY	
TUESDAY	
WEDNESDAY	
THURSDAY	
FRIDAY	
SATURDAY	
SUNDAY	

Notes
_____
_____
_____
_____
_____
_____
_____
_____
_____
_____
_____
_____
_____
_____
_____

PRIORITIES
◯ _____
◯ _____
◯ _____
◯ _____
◯ _____
◯ _____
◯ _____
◯ _____

WEEKLY
planner

WEEK OF _____

MONDAY

TUESDAY

WEDNESDAY

THURSDAY

FRIDAY

SATURDAY

SUNDAY

Notes

_____
_____
_____
_____
_____
_____
_____
_____
_____
_____
_____
_____
_____
_____
_____
_____

PRIORITIES

○ _____
○ _____
○ _____
○ _____
○ _____
○ _____
○ _____
○ _____

WEEKLY
planner

WEEK OF _____

MONDAY

TUESDAY

WEDNESDAY

THURSDAY

FRIDAY

SATURDAY

SUNDAY

Notes

_____
_____
_____
_____
_____
_____
_____
_____
_____
_____
_____
_____
_____
_____
_____
_____
_____

PRIORITIES

○ _____
○ _____
○ _____
○ _____
○ _____
○ _____
○ _____
○ _____

WEEKLY
planner

WEEK OF _____

Notes

PRIORITIES

- MONDAY
- TUESDAY
- WEDNESDAY
- THURSDAY
- FRIDAY
- SATURDAY
- SUNDAY

MONTH:

REVIEW

ILLNESS MANAGEMENT ★ ★ ★ ★ ★   MOOD ★ ★ ★ ★ ★

HIGHLIGHTS OF THE MONTH

THINGS I LEARNED

THINGS I'M GRATEFUL FOR

WAYS TO IMPROVE NEXT MONTH

November

YEAR:_____

SUNDAY	MONDAY	TUESDAY	WEDNESDAY	THURSDAY	FRIDAY	SATURDAY

Habit Tracker

| Month | | Year | |

HABIT	1	2	3	4	5	6	7	8	9	10	11	12	13	14	15	16	17	18	19	20	21	22	23	24	25	26	27	28	29	30	31

Symptom Tracker

SYMPTOM	1	2	3	4	5	6	7	8	9	10	11	12	13	14	15	16	17	18	19	20	21	22	23	24	25	26	27	28	29	30	31

WEEKLY
planner

WEEK OF _____

MONDAY

TUESDAY

WEDNESDAY

THURSDAY

FRIDAY

SATURDAY

SUNDAY

Notes

_____
_____
_____
_____
_____
_____
_____
_____
_____
_____
_____
_____
_____
_____
_____

PRIORITIES

- ○ _____
- ○ _____
- ○ _____
- ○ _____
- ○ _____
- ○ _____
- ○ _____
- ○ _____

WEEKLY
planner

WEEK OF _____

MONDAY

TUESDAY

WEDNESDAY

THURSDAY

FRIDAY

SATURDAY

SUNDAY

Notes

_____
_____
_____
_____
_____
_____
_____
_____
_____
_____
_____
_____
_____
_____
_____
_____
_____
_____

PRIORITIES

○ _____
○ _____
○ _____
○ _____
○ _____
○ _____
○ _____
○ _____

WEEKLY
planner

WEEK OF _____

MONDAY

TUESDAY

WEDNESDAY

THURSDAY

FRIDAY

SATURDAY

SUNDAY

Notes
_____
_____
_____
_____
_____
_____
_____
_____
_____
_____
_____
_____
_____
_____
_____
_____
_____

PRIORITIES
○ _____
○ _____
○ _____
○ _____
○ _____
○ _____
○ _____
○ _____

WEEKLY
planner

WEEK OF _____

MONDAY

TUESDAY

WEDNESDAY

THURSDAY

FRIDAY

SATURDAY

SUNDAY

Notes

_____
_____
_____
_____
_____
_____
_____
_____
_____
_____
_____
_____
_____
_____
_____
_____

PRIORITIES

○ _____
○ _____
○ _____
○ _____
○ _____
○ _____
○ _____
○ _____

WEEKLY
planner

WEEK OF _____

MONDAY	
TUESDAY	
WEDNESDAY	
THURSDAY	
FRIDAY	
SATURDAY	
SUNDAY	

Notes

_____
_____
_____
_____
_____
_____
_____
_____
_____
_____
_____
_____
_____
_____
_____

PRIORITIES

○ _____
○ _____
○ _____
○ _____
○ _____
○ _____
○ _____
○ _____

MONTH:

REVIEW

ILLNESS MANAGEMENT ★ ★ ★ ★ ★   MOOD ★ ★ ★ ★ ★

HIGHLIGHTS OF THE MONTH

THINGS I LEARNED

THINGS I'M GRATEFUL FOR

WAYS TO IMPROVE NEXT MONTH

December

YEAR: _____

SUNDAY	MONDAY	TUESDAY	WEDNESDAY	THURSDAY	FRIDAY	SATURDAY

Habit Tracker

Month		Year	

HABIT	1	2	3	4	5	6	7	8	9	10	11	12	13	14	15	16	17	18	19	20	21	22	23	24	25	26	27	28	29	30	31

Symptom Tracker

SYMPTOM	1	2	3	4	5	6	7	8	9	10	11	12	13	14	15	16	17	18	19	20	21	22	23	24	25	26	27	28	29	30	31

WEEKLY
planner

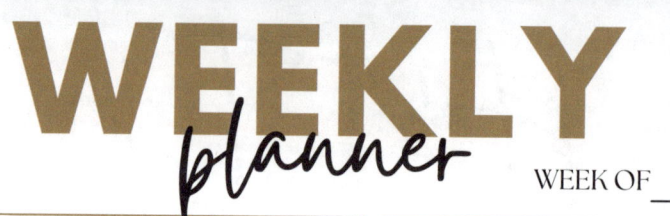

WEEK OF _____

MONDAY

TUESDAY

WEDNESDAY

THURSDAY

FRIDAY

SATURDAY

SUNDAY

Notes

PRIORITIES

WEEKLY
planner

WEEK OF _____

MONDAY	
TUESDAY	
WEDNESDAY	
THURSDAY	
FRIDAY	
SATURDAY	
SUNDAY	

Notes

PRIORITIES

- ○
- ○
- ○
- ○
- ○
- ○
- ○
- ○

WEEKLY
planner

WEEK OF _____

Notes

MONDAY

TUESDAY

WEDNESDAY

THURSDAY

FRIDAY

SATURDAY

SUNDAY

PRIORITIES

WEEKLY *planner*

WEEK OF _____

Notes

PRIORITIES

- MONDAY
- TUESDAY
- WEDNESDAY
- THURSDAY
- FRIDAY
- SATURDAY
- SUNDAY

WEEKLY
planner

WEEK OF _____

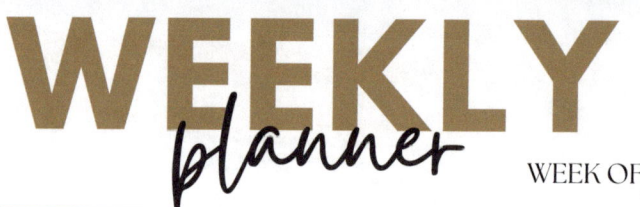

MONDAY

TUESDAY

WEDNESDAY

THURSDAY

FRIDAY

SATURDAY

SUNDAY

Notes

_____
_____
_____
_____
_____
_____
_____
_____
_____
_____
_____
_____
_____
_____
_____
_____

PRIORITIES

○ _____
○ _____
○ _____
○ _____
○ _____
○ _____
○ _____
○ _____

MONTH:

REVIEW

ILLNESS MANAGEMENT ★ ★ ★ ★ ★   MOOD ★ ★ ★ ★ ★

HIGHLIGHTS OF THE MONTH

THINGS I LEARNED

THINGS I'M GRATEFUL FOR

WAYS TO IMPROVE NEXT MONTH

Yearly Review

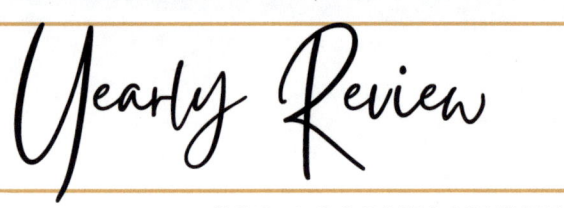

Year

TOP ACCOMPLISHMENTS

HIGHLIGHTS

SETBACKS

THINGS TO LEARN

THINGS TO CHANGE

START

STOP

CONTINUE

NEXT YEAR PRIORITIES

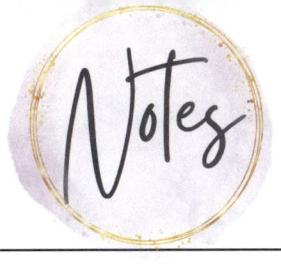

Notes

Notes

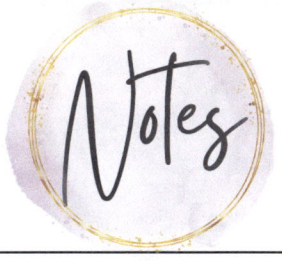

Notes

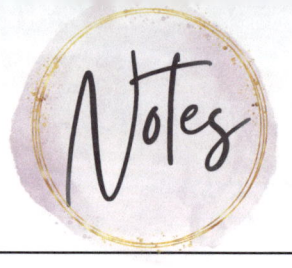

Notes

Notes

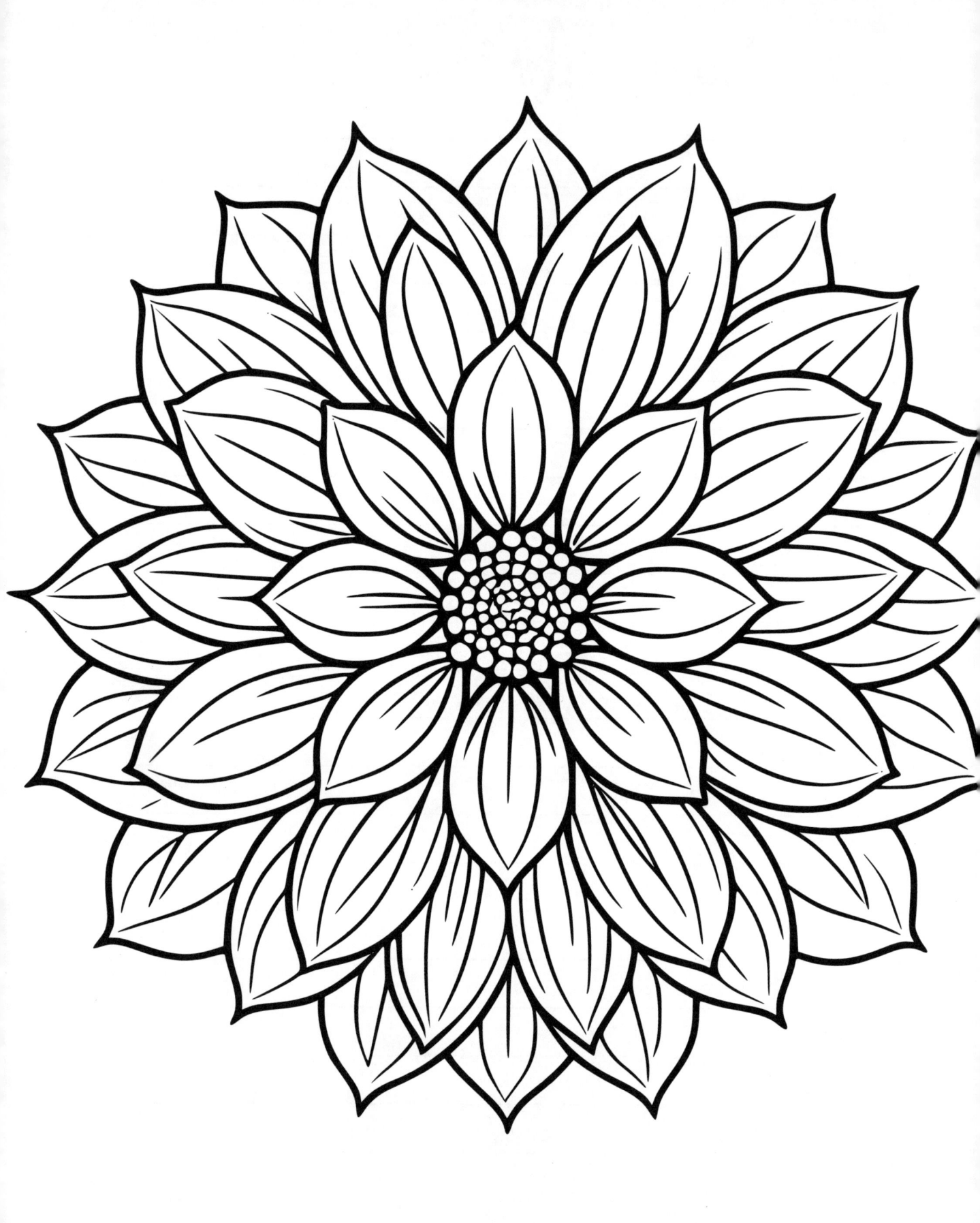

EVERY DAY IS A FRESH START

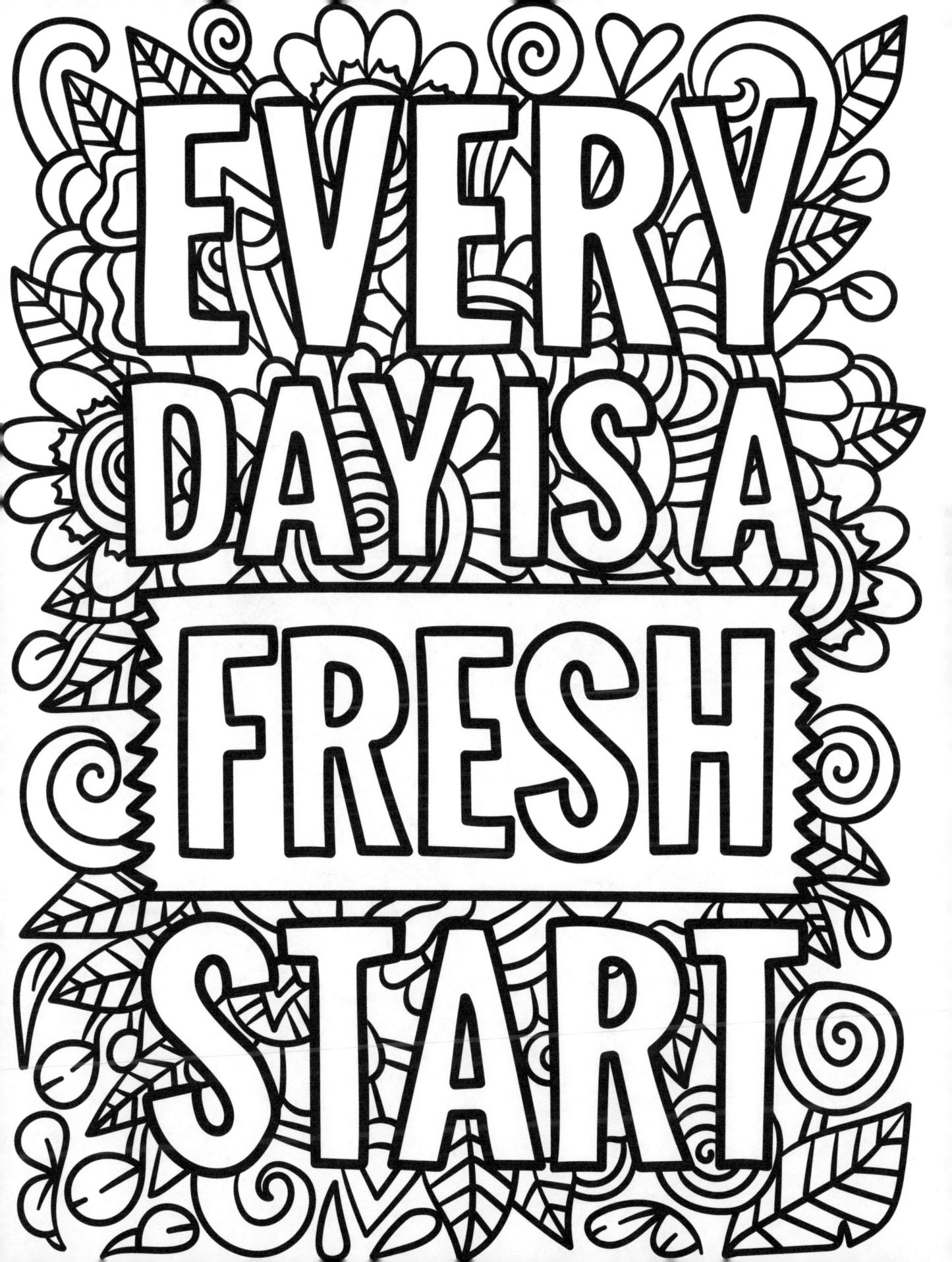

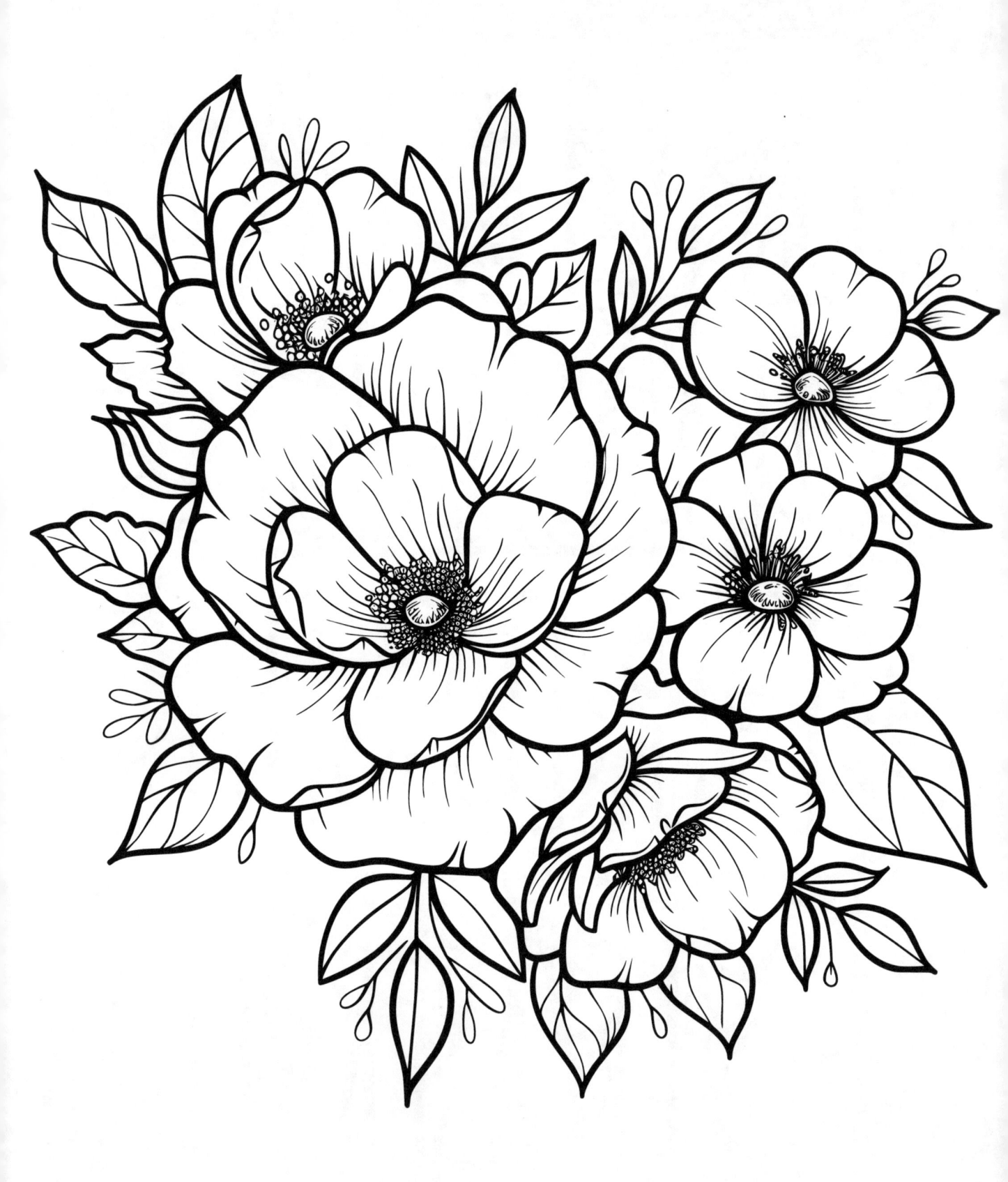

Life is tough but you are

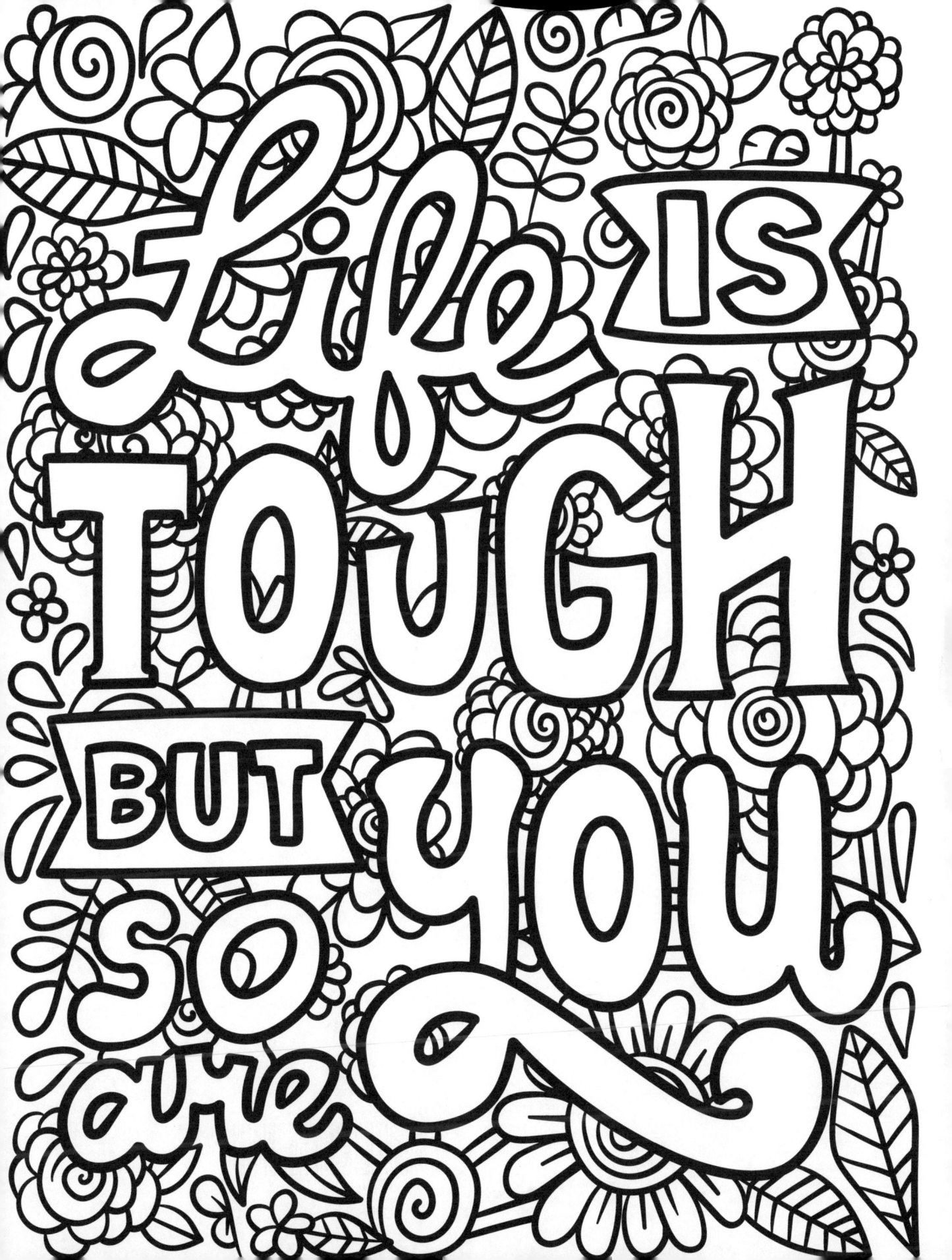

Made in the USA
Columbia, SC
27 November 2024